TIPS ON HOW TO LOSE WEIGHT IN 3 MONTHS

Authored by KG Lim

TABLE OF CONTENTS

What Exactly is a Support System?

Do you know what a support system is? I shall try to explain it in simple terms for you to understand and enjoy the benefits of having one.

Are you feeling alone? Isolated? Helpless? Restless? Unsupported? Confused and Tired? Most probably you are in a situation like all others who need to have friends to talk to or just find people to be able to socialize with and discuss the same concerns as you do. A lot of groups organized to answer a need or respond to a problem are actually forms of what a support system is. People with different types of interests, like religion, music and arts, lifestyle, problems are some examples. A classic example of a support system is your family who knows just what you are going through and is actually there to support you emotionally and psychologically. Your network of friends is also an example of people who know you, love you and are there to support you with your plans especially if it is good for you.
Community organizations are examples of support groups that hope to cater to the need of different social groups in one's living environment similar to school organizations.

Members of one's support system depend on one's choice of people to be affiliated with. They have more or less knowledge of your life and concerns. One's support system could be your very own

friends,   family   members,   classmates,   or acquaintances that
are in the same situation as you are or are concerned with what you are doing or feeling at the given moment.

Members of your own support system actually take the time to be involved with how you respond and handle the situation you are currently in. They actually contribute to your knowledge on the subject from their own wealth of resources as you open yourself up to them. They may often provide you a different perspective on how you see things and could actually give more objective, specific and concrete views. A support group is also a healthy environment to check whether you are on the right track or not. Basically, your own support system provides you the non-material support that you need in whatever circumstances in your life.

Support systems in relation support groups establish contact with persons who share the same concern and interest or are actually sympathetic to the cause through communication. Promotions are done in writing such as invitations and advertisements even on-line. In these ways, support groups and your own support system could go over a wide variety of people from different realities that could help enrich your very own experience in life as you work towards your goals.

Socializing and letting others get to know what you do is an important part of a healthy social and emotional life.

Establish your own support system. There are a lot of things that you can get from having your own support system or support group. You actually get more lasting benefits through them than when you work to achieve your goals all by yourself.

Setting Small Goals as a Constant Motivator

All of us have goals and all of us want to achieve it. If your goal is to lose weight, here are few important things about goals which you should know.

The desire to lose weight and enjoy its benefits would only be materialized with proper action, support and constant motivation.

You heard it right! Without these important elements, your dream of achieving your ideal weight would never come to fruition. In all goals and goal setting, the clarity with what it is you want to have is the primary requirement for the total plan of action. Goals are there to help provide structure and focus in achieving your dream. Each individual who has an idea of what he or she wants can and would gladly do an outline of how his or her life should be lived and where to direct it. Things such as lifetime goals, long-term goals and life-direction courses are means to mapping out how you want to live your life.

But more importantly, lifetime goals are comprised of small and short-term goals set to put you on course towards the end of your quest for success. Some people who have the desire to succeed in achieving their goals do not succeed. Why is this so? People tend to articulate highly abstract and ideal thoughts when it comes to goal setting, forgetting that goals should be attainable, reasonable, time-constrained, concrete and specific. Setting lifetime goals without its accompanying short-term goals would easily sway you from focusing on your goal and spending a lot of your energies to activities that may not be relevant to your cause. Short-term, small goals are helpful to keep your ship on sail towards the promised benefits of your dreams. These small and helpful goals would constantly remind you of your motivation and reason for wanting to achieve your goal in the end. They are practical tools to slowly realize your long-term plans.

Basically, small goals provide you a workable objective that would easily fit into the over-all plan of your generally abstract ideal in the end. Setting small goals is a unique and creative activity of self-expression as you try to sift in and include the factors that are very much relevant to you. Examples of these are your budget, your lifestyle, your work or career, your availability or the actual hours that you can possibly set aside for your routines and your environment as they all play significant roles in your plan to lose weight.

Small goals that may help you achieve your long-term plan may include:

·   Saving a few dollars from buying convenient foods such as fast food and processed goods
·   Including vegetables and fruits in your meal everyday

·   Maintaining proper posture wherever you are as it burns a small amount of calories
·   Getting enough sleep everyday

·   A minute or two to practice proper breathing especially in the morning after waking up

·   Setting thirty minutes to an hour to relax and release tension by doing your daily exercise

·   Imaging yourself with the body size that you want in a few moments everyday or as you start your mentally
    conditions one to maintain the train of thoughts that are essential to achieving the thought

Why Almost all Diets Fail

Although dieting provides a lot of benefits to people like you, there can also be a hundred reasons why diets fail.

I know this news sound so heartless, but lend me your eyes as you continue reading. Mostly, it all depends on the person who is committed to the activity. You already know that dieting is not a form of a magic trick that will easily turn anyone into a handsome prince or a beautiful princess , you need to exert hard work. I'm sure you can do it.

Since there are other usual occasions that add to the drama, it is quite normal to find other people give up on their dream to lose weight or at least live a healthier life. You may just be one of these persons. Did you know that learning why diets fail can actually help you target the solutions for your own dieting problems? Being able to understand the causes of diet failures will aid you to make preventive measures so as not to go into the same pit of despair. I came up with a few reasons why almost all diets fail:

1.   You Simply Don't Believe In It
·   It may sound childish and petty to you, but you have to admit it. I am also guilty of this sometimes. Everyone who goes into a new diet plan experiences that stage of inevitable doubt. What if it doesn't work out? What if you end up gaining more weight? What if this diet is not for you? Instead of asking all these "what if's", why not ask yourself why you don't believe in it. I'm sure you'll be quite surprised to find

out that doubt comes from your own feeling of pessimism. When you know that there is no chance in hell for you to keep up with your diet plan, then it will simply not happen. You have to remember that all things you do in life are dependent on your points of view and your perspectives. This is also why it is important to be positive and believe that it will all work out. I know this sounds too hard at first. In may be in a matter of weeks or months before you start seeing changes, but hey, at least you know there would be some.

2. You've Tried It Before

·   Yes, you failed. Should we get over that idea and start things anew? There would always be times when you would feel as if you are in for a failure since you have been to the same situation and saw yourself going for the dumpsters.

Well hear this, it is high time you change that about yourself! I know you may have miserably failed during the past while keeping up with your old diet plan. But that shouldn't stop you from turning that failure into something that will make you prouder in the end? The best thing about recovering from failures is that you are able to prove something to yourself and the other people around you.

4. You Have the Wrong Diet Plan

·   It may be your fault or that of your nutritionist's, but regardless of who made the wrong decision, it is still your diet plan. Own it and do something about it. I have my own share of experiences with a wrong diet plan that caused a lot of topsy-turvy scenarios in my health life. To correct that, I went for a better diet plan. Bear in mind that the only way to correct a wrong diet plan is to go with something that has been proven and tested. I suggest you consult with a nutritionist recommended by a family member or a friend. That way, you know the person who assisted you with the plan is someone who is an expert in the field and can be trusted.

Incorporating Exercise Into Your Daily Life

Did you know that there are a lot of benefits for practicing cardiovascular activities wherever you are and whatever time of the day? I know that you are a busy person, and sometimes there are just a lot of things left to do for everyday. This and a hundred more reasons keep you from going to the gym or reserving a few minutes of your time for cardiovascular exercises. Well, you know what? Cardiovascular activities are important to help strengthen the immune system, and to promote healthier lungs along with other organs in our internal systems. If you are having problems adjusting to your busy schedule at work or has fears on going through strenuous exercises, well my suggestions may be perfect for you. In truth, you do not always need to be in a gym or a fitness center to incorporate a few exercises during your extra time. You can do very simple tasks on a daily basis to help you keep those muscles moving and to make sure that smooth blood circulation is present in your body. Trust me on this, dear. Here are some examples:

1. Walking Your Way to a Healthy Life
·   As much as possible, take advantage of the opportunity to walk from one place to another. I know this may sound very stressful at first since a lot of people do not like the idea of walking, especially when they are in a hurry. But come on! If you need to get to another place fast, then try brisk walking. You can get a lot of exercise by simply walking from

your car to the entrance of a building. You may want to try parking a few spaces farther from the building entrance to give yourself more chances of building up with your exercises. I'm positive you'll feel great about this! Naturally, with your parking space farther from the entrance than usual, you will not only be able to do a bit of cardiovascular stints, you will also be able to easily spot a parking space by the time you arrive at work.

2.   Taking the Stairs to a New You
·   That's right. Enough of the elevators and escalators! I know you love them, but it is time to use your own feet to climb up those steps. I am a fan of technology, but I'm a bigger aficionado of keeping myself   in tiptop shape. Why don't you give yourself a break from all the slacking and boredom? Find adventure by using the stairs when going to the fifth floor or the rooftop. This is not only an excellent way for you to shed off a few pounds, it will also keep your respiratory and circulatory systems in a stable pattern of blood and oxygen exchange. Isn't that wonderful?

3.   Time to Do Your "Homework"
·   No, not those written assignments from your professors. I mean house chores and learning how to work in the garden and your kitchen. I know you may not be good in cooking or gardening, so make yourself useful by cleaning up the house. Working on some important house chores will not only help you incorporate exercise in your daily life, it will also

benefit everyone inside the house. Living in a clean and safe home is the best way to live a healthy life.

Benefits of a Support System

If achieving goals and realizing your dreams are encouraged through perseverance, persistence and enough motivation, why would you need to have a support system along the way? What is so special about having a support system? What would a support system give you? There are a lot to know about support system.

In anything you do for yourself as you realize your plans or goals, there may come a time when you need to slow down and check whether what you are doing is in keeping with the over-all plan or not. Losing weight for example is not immune to the many chances of being distracted, once in a while, by personal concerns and setbacks, not to mention the many questions you may have as you develop your own program and routine.

Consulting a professional about your plan is a good way to start your own exercise program but having friends along the way adds more to the fun and experience of your own journey. Since friends and family members are always there when you need to, talking out your plans and concerns to them add meaning to the whole experience especially when you need positive thoughts in working your way.

A support system is a network of friends, family members, acquaintances who know what is happening to you and provide you the non-material support that you need to realize your personal dreams and goals. This support system is established as one takes the opportunities to be open to the people who can directly influence the way you live or direct your life.

Your own support system is like a mirror where you can actually see yourself as becoming fitter or not in the course of your plans. There are a lot of benefits in having your own support system. Benefits of having a support system include:

- A safe environment for personal reflection and sharing.
- A place to air out personal concerns and worries
- Helpful answers to your very own questions
- Give a realistic assessment of your own goals
- Could provide you with a healthy self-doubt by presenting other possibilities to your concern.
- The sense of enjoyment in working with a group of people who value what you do.
- Encourage you to persevere
- Remind you of your goals
- Help motivate you when you are slacking off
- Check your thoughts
- Allow you to socialize and meet people
- Provides opportunities to direct one's concern outside of one's self once in a while.
- Give suggestions that you may have overlooked

These benefits and more are available to you as you develop and establish your very own support system. It does not need to be anything special with specific requirements and 'to do' lists. All you need to do is consider who are the people in your life that are more than willing to help you in making your dream come true. Who knows? These people might be as excited to change their lives through proper diet and healthy living just as you do.

You can take this as daily doses in making you a better person, both inside and out. I am very confident that you will be able to witness more changes in your life in the years to come. At first, things may be difficult for you since this system requires a lot of focus, discipline and determination. However, I know for a fact that you can do it, so do not give up. If you feel like you are on the verge of giving up on your course to losing weight, take the time to relax your mind and muscles for a moment. Sometimes, the body also needs a little time to rest and to recuperate their strength.

1. Keep on Trying
·   Having set the right goals, I am certain that you will find it easier to find ways to become slimmer in just a matter of days. Should you find any of our suggestions quite unsuccessful for you, do not give up. The key to losing weight is to never stop trying so just keep doing all the exercises and be posted in the schedules of your dietary   plan   to   achieve maximum results. If you have already been doing so, I would like to express my utmost gratitude for your trust and confidence in our output. I know that greater results will flourish in your life even more if you continue to try and do not let any means or

obstacles get in the way to make you feel good about yourself.

2.   Give Yourself the Time to Let Loose
·   As what I have said in the beginning, there will be trying times. You will feel exhausted, hopeless, and at worse, frantic. But to do not let these emotions bring you down, instead treat them as stepping stones to achieving the new you. If you need a few minutes to relax after your workout plan, then give yourself that right. If you know you are working hard, you also deserve to rest. As with all parts in goal-setting, you need to set aside a time for yourself to simply relax and enjoy the benefits of the course we have set up for you. Do not be afraid to give yourself an opportunity to be free and to let loose.

3.   Take it One Step at a Time
·   No one's rushing you to lose weight or to immediately achieve your goals, so do not overstress yourself. Just take things one step at a time, and I know you will be able to do things right in your own time. Bear in mind that each person has a different way of dealing with things in life, so do not be too bothered. If you do not get positive results right away, just go try again and take things as they come. Do not get ahead of yourself by forcing things to come to you. Benefits of the program will come in naturally. So just wait, and do what you have to do.

Benefits of Dieting

You may be one of those people who have been desperately trying to lose weight their entire lives. Lucky for you, I have found your new best friend in dieting. Did you know that dieting provides a lot of benefits to an individual's life? It does not only improve one's outlook on a physical level, this also strengthens the mental and emotional state of a person by helping you feel good about what you eat. I am sure you'll be thrilled to find out that by having a healthy diet, a person is able to give their bodies the right amount of nutrition and energy needed for everyday. Without observing the proper diet, a lot of people may be subjected to malnutrition and may not be able to perform at their best, regardless of their known capabilities. I'm concerned you may be one of these people. For me to help you out, here are some of the proven benefits of dieting:

1. Prevention of Diseases
· Cardiovascular diseases are the leading causes of deaths for every year. Are you sure you're eating the right food to help nourish your heart and blood flow? Problems may arise concerning your health if you do not take my advice. Fruits and vegetables, for instance, reduce the risk of stroke and other diseases in the circulatory system. With the right balance of food groups in your diet, and with the presence of fruits and vegetables, you can expect better results coming from your annual preventive checkups. I'll be happy to learn that you are doing ways to help prevent the growth of other diseases

and its symptoms by use of the nutrients that will aid your body to strengthen its immune system.

2. More Focus and Less Stress

· A lot of people battle stress and unconsciousness everyday; I too am a victim of these two. You may well be one of these people. Let us find ways together for you to prevent such emotions. Focus on the things that you eat and find a way to make your diet better. If you are already following a strict diet and you seem not to be able to concentrate on anything at work, due to the feeling weariness and fatigue, do yourself a favor and look into the things that you eat. Let me help you lessen those nauseating feelings experienced by both our bodies due to lack of certain nutrients in our system. Making sure that the right balance of all essential vitamins is present in your daily diet, will certainly help alleviate stress.

3. Feel Good About Yourself

· What more reason are you asking for? Everyone wants to feel good about themselves and how they carry themselves in front of other people. Do yourself that favor by eating the right food. Having a well-balanced diet will eventually help you reach your desired weight, making you feel better and more comfortable with your body. Even those with perfect body figures, still maintain their respective diets so as to make sure that they have a balanced physique. Do not let other people solely enjoy what you can also have. Give yourself a break from all those unnecessary meals and focus on eating healthier foods. If people see that you feel good about yourself, it will also be easier for them to hang out with you as they reciprocate that positive glow. I know you can do it.

What Are the Benefits of Supplements?

What Are Supplements?
With the worldwide mania for bodybuilding, it is undeniable that hundreds if not thousands of body building products sprouted like mushrooms—all claiming to sustain the body's needs and all of which are for better health. The most popular of all are body building supplements that include memory teasers, growth stimulants, mood enhancers, and dietary supplements. Perhaps you do not know that all of these products are made to improve your health and boost your stamina. Supplements are made to provide what your body needs. As a bodybuilder, you are burning more fats and calories than a normal individual. For this reason, you need to take more vitamins, minerals, and other substances so as not to compromise your health.

The Benefits of Food Supplements
Allow me to discuss basic things about organic supplements. Organic supplements are a lot more concentrated than normal food and vitamins. These supplements come mostly in tablet form and should be taken daily. The dosage also may vary for every user depending on the weight, the body building work out plans, and the daily routines. These supplements are produced under certain standards. They normally come from plants and are extracted to a concentrate so the body will get more than it can normally get in normal eating.

Many people simply do not have the time to prepare food that is ideal for their body building routines. Did you know that these people also work and they simply will not have the time or perhaps the energy to prepare the food they need? One of the benefits of food supplements is that it gives you the ability to nourish yourself adequately without having to think about the ordeal you have to go through in preparing ideal meals for the day.

Supplements also ensure that you receive adequate nutrition for the calories you lost during your work out. A normal person may have enough nutrition from the normal food he is eating. However, there is a big difference for people who are into body building. As you lift more weights, you tear your muscles apart and the activities of your body to repair these damaged tissues is way beyond a normal person's. In short, your body is working about twice as hard as a normal person. Due to this, what you normally eat will not be enough.

Popular Food Supplements: Weight Loss Tea and Acai Berry

Perhaps the most popular of all supplements are the weight loss tea and acai berry. For thousands of years, tea has been claimed as a plant that has healing powers, that it does not do any damage to the body. It was proven to help the body develop its immune system and therefore get rid of potential diseases. It has antioxidants that slow degenerative diseases from entering the body. The main thing

about tea is that it has about 30-40% of polyphenols.
According to doctors, the body needs about 300-400 milligrams if this substance in a day.

Acai Berry, on the other hand, has high levels of proteins. These are like the protein that we get form eggs. These proteins lower cholesterol levels and thus helps the body become a lot more fit and healthy.

What are Supplements

Do you have your own bottle of supplements? I do! Supplements are often distinguished as a type of drug or food product however, they are actually not. Did you know that legal definitions have been scribed regarding the contents of supplements and what they can do for human beings . The United States Food and Drug Administration or the FDA upholds strong regulations on how the manufacturing of supplements must adhere to specific functions different from other medications sold in drugstores. Quite a mouthful, huh? Well, supplements can come in different forms and uses. I'm quite confused about them too at first. But finding more about them just makes me feel healthier and more secured about my lifestyle. I'm sure you'll make great use of them too! There are supplements that come in a form of a vitamin for everyday, providing people like you and me countless sources of energy. I was also able to find out those supplements' contents are minerals that are essential to the human body.

If you must know, there is already a growing population of people who use supplements for herbal needs, which are often relative to specific medical functions. Since I also dream of losing weight, supplements have also helped me in achieving my dream vital stats. Whatever your reason is for consuming supplements, it is important for you to know what they do for your body and overall health.

.

What the Body Needs

·   I know not everyone has all the luxury in the world to keep a close watch on our health. But hey, why don't you   give it a try? To save us both some of our most precious time, supplements find a way to keep us healthy. Although a lot of people may be eating three meals a day and following strict dietary plans from their nutritionists, you have to admit that they are not always a hundred percent sure that they have all the essential nutrients present in their body. In order to help our bodies defend themselves from diseases and other harmful symptoms, supplements provide us with all the essential vitamins and minerals our body needs.

·   Creating that Balance
·   If your dietary plan does not work for you, your body has no other choice but to rely on whatever mineral or   nutrient is present in your body. This may sound as the saddest truth in life, even I couldn't believe it at first.

     Did you also know that supplements allow your body to create a balance among all systems thereby ensuring that all meals we consume on a daily basis are going through a wide process of nutrient breakdown to help disseminate in different bodily systems? Once this happens, you can expect each system inside your body to function more properly and to avoid the risk of us getting sick. I just find this to be an excellent opportunity for us both!

·   Feel Better Whatever You Do

· I know you find yourself easily getting exhausted from work, which may be caused by your unstable health. Let me help you understand that supplements can keep you going and can assure you all the strength you need to get by everyday. These supplements will help provide your body all sources of optimal health. You will not only feel healthy, but supplements will also help you feel better about everything you do. I know it will just make you feel the extremely well about your health. Trust me on that! Regardless if you have been working too late at night or if you are having a hard time catching up on sleep, you will be able to find other means to keep yourself focused and healthy. Did you also know that some supplements also have the ability to make you lose weight if and in case you have extra pounds you want to shed off?

Ideas On How to Create a Support System

I'll tell you about one important trick on getting more active with exercise and diet through a support system. I will answer why they are necessary and some of its benefits.

The importance of having your own support system gradually shows itself as you move forward in achieving your goals. This may sometimes come up in times of stress, lack of motivation, negative self-talk and unnecessary worries that you encounter as you progress in your own program. Your own support system provides you the invaluable help to get you moving on the proper road to succeed with your plans.

But how do we start a support system? Who are included? And where do we find such people to help us?

A support system is a network or group of persons who are personally involved with each other by a common and often shared interest or advocacy providing individuals non-material support and help through communication.

Members of a support system could be one's friends, classmates, acquaintances, officemates, family members and anyone who are willing to be involved with you and with what you do. In a similar manner, you become part of a support system when you personally get yourself into participating and helping your friends achieve their own goals or the group's causes. People who could be part of your support system could be anyone you personally know but may just be waiting for someone who could articulate the desire. Therefore, it is important that you make yourself known and your thoughts articulated. If you want to lose those extra pounds and look sexy for your loved ones and friends then speak it out before you lose the chance to start early on.

Make yourself heard, make sure you have your own goals with you. Discuss it with friends and invite them to join you in your own program. Spread the word and invite family members and relatives. Usually, the most ideal support system is the one who has deeper knowledge or experience with you as they tend to be more helpful in giving you concrete and objective suggestions.

Write! Sometimes writing is more effective at communications than oral ones especially if the distance crosses borders. People could easily sympathize with you if they hear you through your own testimonies.

Walk the talk. People who actually see you realize your goals are more likely to be interested with what is going on with you. This may encourage them to participate. Encourage people to lead a healthier lifestyle. Generally, health belongs to the higher level in the hierarchy of values so people would express concern about it eventually. Advertise the benefits of losing weight. This strategy actually works in two ways. As you attract people to do what you do and value, you are actually repeating for yourself the very things that you need to remember. Learn more about the topic or do research. As you study the subject, you may meet people along the way who share the same interest as you do.

Finally, the most basic tip in having your own support system is to socialize. It is never too late to have new friends as you keep the old ones.

What Should You Look for in a Workout Plan?

Defining Workout Plans
Let me tell you that for a lot of gym enthusiasts, a workout plans not an entirely new concept, especially for those who have personal trainers. However, this may sound vague and new to people who are just starting with body building. A workout plan is basically a road map to completing and ensuring the success of your physical regimen. You see, lifting weights and taking pills and body supplements will not do you any good if you do not a well defined plan on what you want to achieve and improve on your body. A workout plan will contain the exercises that you will do, how many times they need to be done, how many times a week, what food supplements you need to take, and what your diet should be. In summation, this is a combination of everything that needs to get accomplished to reach your goal, whether it is to increase in muscle size, tone the body, gain weight or lose it.

The Benefits of Having a Work out Plan
As mentioned earlier, lifting weights is not just about competing the exercise, there has to be a goal n why this is being done. Each exercise has an equivalent amount of effort that needs to be acted upon. Also, exercises are divided into categories depending on the part of the body that you need to improve. Let me tell you that the good thing about workout plans is that you will have a set of exercises that will target the specific areas of your body that you need to improve.

Workout plans will give you the quality of exercise that will also yield quality results. Without this, you will just be wasting your time and energy. On top of this, a workout plan will also help you save money because your body building activities and supplementary intake and dietary plans are all synergized. A workout plan will prevent you from getting physically burned out and getting over exercised. When this happens, you reduce the gains from your workout. You spend more and you gain less.

What to Look for in a Workout Plan
Did you know that the first thing you need to look for is the goal? How much calories will you lose in each exercise?
How much fat will you get rid of? Second, you need to see how long the plan will last and when you can expect to see the results. You cannot keep on doing the same exercise without knowing when to see the results. Next, you need to check the alternative exercises available. If you are performing a cardio workout, then you should have at least two types of exercises. This should also include the repetitions number of minutes that you need to perform the exercise.

Truth About ABS
Perhaps you may have heard of this dynamic approach to reducing abdominal fats. In a classical perspective, the only ways to reduce abdominal fats is to do sit-ups or exercises that strain the abdominal area. This new approach is globally sweeping the

body building world because of its radical approach in which you need to identify the cause of having a fat stomach before working on it. This is a practical approach that ensures a guaranteed approach for those who want to get rid of abdominal fats.

What to Look for in a Diet

Well, I know you may be one of those people who desperately fail in keeping their own dietary plans. Have you tried to check what to look for in a diet? Maybe not, but I'm here to help you out. You know that there are a lot of well known diets supported by celebrities and well respected nutritionists that can help an individual live a healthier lifestyle.

However, did you know that not all these are compatible with every body makeup and composition? It is essential to combine the right eating habits as well as a good dietary plan to help a person maintain the most optimum weight for his/her size.

I realized that information related to diets is often very challenging and can contain a lot of difficult tasks so as to reach your ideal physical state. Well, lucky for you I've found a few tips that can help you come up with the best possible diet plan. Check these out:

1.   Know What You Must Avoid
·   Before knowing what to look for, you have to know what you must avoid. Knowing what you must not eat will help you in looking for the best possible plan to aid in giving you the perfect health. Did you know that a lot of people, especially those who have high blood sugar level, need to tone down on cholesterol intake? You may want to keep a close watch on adding food groups that are rich in carbohydrates as you formulate your dietary

scheme. As much as possible, keep away from fats. I highly discourage these as inclusions in dietary plans, and so do other well known nutritionists.

2.   The Essence of Small Servings

·   I know you hate minimal servings of food, but it's high time you know that this can help you in getting the right diet. The best diet is always the one that serves you the least amount of servings. Of course, that does not necessarily mean you have to eat really small dosage even if you incredibly hungry. It means keeping a well-balanced meal.

If you aim to lose weight, less is always more. I know it sounds difficult, but think about the benefits at the end of the day. For instance, while eating dinner, you may want to take a pass on second servings. Try to limit your meals to only one serving of food. That way, you will be able to train your body to be contented in eating less.

3.   The Hearty Meals

·   Did you also know that the most effective diet is the one that keeps three meals a day? These diets include breakfast, lunch and dinner. I know this to be the most perfect dietary plan! Breakfast, of all three, is the most important since this is the main source of energy for your everyday activities. If you must now, there are also dietary plans that go as far as to letting you have five meals a day. But remember what I told you, "Having smaller servings and yet ore chances to eat will help you keep up with your diet by not feeling hungry all the time."

Get Active with Exercising

An easy way to get started with your goal of losing weight is to do cardiovascular exercises.

Cardiovascular exercises are one of the important forms of exercises that one must incorporate into one's exercise program. They prevent the risks of acquiring coronary heart disease as they strengthen the lungs and the heart. These exercises work on the larger mass of muscles in the body such as the legs and the arms. Most exercises are aerobic in nature which means oxygen is delivered more thoroughly in the different parts of the body which is necessary to burn calories.

I'll tell you of some simple exercises for beginners.

A lot of exercise programs are available for beginners. One may actually consult a trainer for the type of program that he or she may have. But there are free and simple ways to do exercise aside from going to the gym or consulting a professional about your weight loss program. Doing simple exercises are sometimes more than enough to cover the expenses you would have for professional training. One just have to be active and persistent to do simple forms of exercises to get as much result as going to the gym pr buying expensive equipment.

A basic requirement in doing any form of exercise is to have the proper posture. Correct posture of standing, sitting and moving your hands could burn calories in little amounts. Start straightening that back of yours and avoid slouching. A mental exercise of awareness about how you compose your self may just be a helpful addition to your daily exercise.

You do not have to automatically go to the gym to start burning fat and lose weight. Simple cardiovascular exercises like walking, cycling, jogging, swimming, rowing and jumping are easy to start with depending on your convenience. Walking is considered as the easiest cardiovascular exercise because all of us have to get moving at any time of the day. The activity is also without doubt, one which covers most of a person's lifetime. You can find ways to do exercise as you go through your daily activities.

Some of the simple ways that encourage cardiovascular activities are:

·   Parking your car a few blocks from your office and walking the remaining distance should help you burn calories and strengthen the muscles of your legs

·   Getting down a few blocks from your house or office and walking the remaining distance does the same effect as the previous

·   Riding the bicycle to your work if possible helps you stretch those arm and leg muscles

· If you have a pool in your house or near you, you may spend thirty minutes for a few lapses

· Walk your pet or your dog around the neighborhood. This is quite an easy and enjoyable task to do.

· Do jump ropes in your backyard for at least a few minutes. This increases your heart activity that stimulates the need for more oxygen.

· Jog around the house or the neighborhood

· Do stretching and squats as you wake up in the morning

Best Wishes and Encouragement

Although things may be rough in the beginning, I give you my warmest blessings to achieving your goals. Please do not be bothered by things that may come your way as you go through exercises, dieting and supplements. Just remember that theses are all part of the process in renewing yourself and making yourself healthier and getting that slimmer figure. I know that wishing you the best and encouraging you to challenge yourself will not only help you to arrive at better results, it will make you a better person at the end of the day. To help you get by the entire course, I wish you nothing but these three things:

1.   I wish you strength and endurance.
·   You will need all the strength that you need to keep on fighting. I don't mean to discourage you in any way, but we all know that there will be tough times throughout this course. Since dieting and workout do not always give you optimum results in a matter of minutes, you have to be patient and to keep that strength within you to carry out your exercises even if you are starting to feel hopeless. These are all part of the challenges that will come your way, but do not let this ruin your strength and endurance to be better at what you do. You will need these two to keep on fighting and to complete the entire course we have lined up for you. So, just hang in there. I believe you'll make it through.

2.   I wish you discipline.

·   Temptation will come, that's for sure. I'm sure you'll find a time when you feel that getting out of your dietary plan and pursuing other unhealthier goals in life is the best way to go. You need the right amount of discipline to keep you going, and I'm confident that you'll do just that. I know that by wishing you discipline, you will be able to make yourself more effective in getting things on track and achieving the goals you have set from the very beginning. Be disciplined and work harder each day to bring about the best results you have ever imagined.

3.   I encourage you to challenge yourself.

·   Yes, you read it right. Challenge yourself. What better way to make yourself more pleasing in your own eyes than to challenge yourself to keep on getting better? The key to achieving more things in less time is to continue in challenging yourself and believing that you will be able to get by any challenges with great ease. If you know that your workout regime is starting to become easy for you, then double up the exercises. I've had my own shares of challenges, believe me. Bear in mind that challenges are always a huge part of all diet plans and exercise schedules, so make good use of them. Just keep on challenging yourself and you may see better results at the end of the day.

After going through the entire course, I am very positive in the end results and we know that you will be able to achieve all your goals. I wish you nothing but the best in your venture to getting that slimmer body and healthier physique. Never give up on your goals to become slimmer and more beautiful.

Make Sure You have All Your Goals Set and are Following an Outline

There are a number of things that you should have done by now. I know that you may be having a hard time focusing on the entire course, but I also know that you will be able to slowly get the hang of things. If you are not sure if you have made every step in creating a healthier and better new you, I created this checklist for you. It's a list of the things you have gone through throughout the entire course:

1. Setting Goals
·   That's right. You now have set a vision for yourself on what you want to achieve in every aspect of your being. You know the benefits of goal-setting and what it can do for you. If you haven't done this yet, take note of all your aspirations and drive yourself to create ways on how to achieve them. I must remind you to make smaller goals so as to help you cross the finish line the soonest possible time. You already know the dangers that plague you in case goals are not set in life.

2. Support Group
·   It may be your friends, family members or special someone. I'm sure you have lots of supporters out You must know that it is important to include a lot of people to support you in your endeavors.

Having a steady support group will help you get motivated in achieving the goals that you have set in life.

Help them help you, and you will surely feel that achieving your goals has never been any easier.

3. Get Active

·   Incorporating exercises in your daily life will not only help you have added movement to your physical body. I'm just positive that getting you active will optimize your lifestyle in every way possible! It will help you give yourself the time to exercise especially at this time when you have no time to go to the gym. Take the time in going up the stairs or parking far from your building entrance to give you an opportunity to stretch those muscles.

4. Diets

·   What more can I say about diets? We all know that keeping a well-balanced diet will not only help nourish your body, but will release that glow within you that you rightfully deserve. As you have learned with me, eating the heartiest meals everyday will ensure the right amount of nutrients needed by your bodily systems. I'm sure you remember that dieting is also the main key to losing weight.

5. Supplements

·   If you don't have the time to give your body all the nutrients, minerals and vitamins that it needs, then it's good that you have learned the facts about supplements with me. Incorporate it in your daily lives to make you stronger and healthier. Try the products that I have recommended to you and witness the benefits of supplements yourself.

6.   Workout Plans

.   If you have all the time in the world to do it, work out. It provides you countless benefits, which should motivate you to start stretching those muscles. Get that six pack abs by following the regime that I helped you out with. Working out will increase cardiovascular strength and will prevent the possibilities of you getting heart-related diseases.

Workout Plan Recommendations-Truth About Abs

Defining a Workout plan

There are a lot of things that a would-be body builder must consider before getting into it. First off, he should have a workout plan, something that may sound new for a newbie. A workout plan is nothing more than a roadmap that needs to be followed to achieve the desired results of body building. Did you know that this contains the exercises that need to be performed, including the diet and that this also contains the number of repetitions that a person needs for each exercise, the body supplements that need to be taken, the amount of calories that will be lost for each exercise, the equipment that need to be used for each exercise, the number of minutes each exercise need to be performed, and all that? Essentially, this is a very detailed plan for a gym enthusiast.

Why Use a Workout Plan?

Without a workout plan, you are likely to get burned out and over exercised without getting the desired results that you are aiming for. With a workout plan, you can calculate how much calories you will lose and you can manage your activities based on your goals. You can also manage your daily diet and your intake of body building and food supplements. Using a workout plan allows you to plan ahead since you can predict your gains using calculators. You see, not all people have the same needs.

Each person has specific needs in terms of calories and each person has a maximum limit of what he can do in his exercise regimen n a daily basis. What is effective for one person may bring failure to another. Each workout plan is crafted for the individual, tailor fit to his needs.

What You Need to Look Out For

I, for one, will tell you that the first thing you need to look for in a workout plan is the exercise activities. Make sure that these exercises are targeting the specific muscle groups that you need to improve. There is no use doing an exercise that will not improve the specific muscles you want to grow. Next, look if there is a timetable for the exercise. The time table should contain the number of minutes to be spent for each exercise and for how long in terms of weeks or months. I also think you should also see the results you should expect when reviewing a workout plan.

Truth About Abs

Even though it is true that the internet is filled with scammers, there are still a few products and approaches out there that are guaranteed to bring satisfactory results to gym and body building enthusiasts, especially in terms of reducing the fats in the abdominal area, called the abs. This is one of the most challenging of all physical fitness buffs. Essentially, the approach is not to do exercises right away. The way this works is to first identify what causes the abs to grow big.

Why are there fats in there that do not seem to get lost? Once the reason is identified, such as parasites, only then will one start to work out.

What is a Workout Plan?

Workout Plan Defined
Essentially, a workout plan in the world of bodybuilding is about combining the exercises you need to accomplish and for how long. This is to make sure that the activities you do will not be put to waste. Workout plans contain what parts of your body will be developed and what will be the expected results. Are you aware that these plans also include what kinds of equipment to use and what the activities are for? These plans also include your dietary plans on a day by day or meal by meal basis. Ideally, plans like this should have a minimum of six weeks coverage. This timetable contains either a daily or week set of exercises that need to be performed depending on the goal. Not all workout plans are the same. These plans are based on your goal for body building and in most cases, these plans are tailor fit to what an individual can do and what he wants to achieve.

The Benefits
Did you know that the main benefit of a workout plan is that you will have a goal and a timetable? You must realize that working out in a gym without any plans at all will not lead you to your goal. With a workout plan, it is true that you are organized and you are following a systematized way of being fit and healthy. Aside from targeting specific areas of your body
for the workout, you will also have a set of defined meals that will back-up your workout regimen. Your

work out plan will contain how many repetitions you need to do for each exercise and the series or order in which these exercises need to be done. This means that your activities are planned carefully to what your body can do. This prevents you from having a physical burnout.

Recommendations and What to Look for in a Workout plan

If you do not have a personal trainer, you must know what a work out plan should have. To begin with, you need to identify what parts of your body you want to grow. Of course, you first need to set a goal. Ask yourself, why are you working out? One you have defined your goals, you are ready to create your own workout plan.

In any workout plan, you need to look for the result. If it is extra muscle that you need, then you need to see that the exercise you are doing will result the extra muscle that you need in the right place. For example, there is no need to do sit-ups if you want to develop your triceps. You also need to make sure that your workout plan shows you how many repetitions should be completed and for how many minutes.

The Truth About ABS

This is a growing popular product or approach regarding working out the abdominal muscles. This approach eradicates classical approaches for developing the abs for both men and women. A lot of trainers claim that sit-ups and food supplements will be enough to get the six-pack abs that you want. This new approach is different in a way that it identifies the source of fat present in your abs. Once this source is identified, only then will you be able to develop a foolproof workout plan.

Supplement Recommendations

Supplements Defined

Admittedly, almost everybody has gone bonkers about health and body building. Due to this, you may have seen a sudden proliferation of body building gyms, food supplements, and all that. What with all these, you of course, should know better that the numbers you want to see are the right weight on the scale, not your name included in bad statistics of body building gone wrong. Did you know that food supplements are made not only for body building enthusiasts. The idea behind food supplements is that these are concentrated forms of nutrients for people who need them. For example, you might need more protein than a normal individual because you work out, then you need to take food supplements rich in protein to cover up your protein and calorie loss after your workout. Some people need food supplements specifically designed for the liver because they might be experiencing liver problems.

Importance of Food Supplements

Food supplements are designed to target specific nutritional needs. As you well know, we have an ideal food group and what is also called a food pyramid. There are five food groups for this pyramid:
· Meat, eggs, fish, dry beans, poultry, and nuts
· Milk, cheese, and yogurt
· Vegetables
· Fruits
· Bread, cereal, rice, and pasta

Let me tell you that you should take more of the food at the bottom of the pyramid and less of sweets and food rich in cholesterol. The problem is, one cannot have adequate time to identify what exactly among these food groups he should take more. If you are working, I doubt it that you will have the time to prepare your meals as recommended by your trainer. Besides, it is an ordeal looking at ingredients and calculating your nutritional needs. As an alternative, you have food supplements out there. All you need is to pop a tablet and off you go.

Weight Loss Tea
Perhaps the most popular non-tablet and non-pill form of food supplement is the weight loss tea. It is not a secret that for hundreds or even thousands of years, tea has been considered as a health drink. Now, there are hundreds of brands out there in the market in various forms: liquid, powder, hot and cold, etc... Tea contains about 40% of polyphenols. These
are substances that our body needs to fight bacteria and other harmful substances that cause diseases. According to statistics, our body needs about 400 milligrams of polyphenols everyday.

Acai Berry
Perhaps you are not aware that the other very popular form of food supplement is the acai berry. Acai berries have very high levels of protein content. Research shows that these berries have more proteins than egg whites. For many body builders, protein is an essential nutrient to have since the

muscles are burning fats and calories, add to this the wear and tear of the muscles during the session. Acai berries also have antioxidants that ward off cancer. Of course, no antioxidant will allow you to be immortal. It's just that antioxidants will prolong your life and having them is better than nothing at all.